I0696302

The Power of Colors: How they affect Mental Wellbeing

Colors are an essential part of our lives, surrounding us wherever we go. But beyond their aesthetic appearance, colors have a profound impact on our mental well-being. For millennia, cultures around the world have attributed symbolic and emotional meanings to different colors, recognizing their power to influence our emotions, our mood and even our mental health. In this text, we will explore the connection between colors and mental well-being, analyzing how colors can influence our emotions and providing insights into how we can harness this knowledge to improve our daily lives.

The Emotional Meaning of Colors: Different colors evoke unique emotions and sensations. For example, blue is often associated with calm and tranquility, while red can evoke intense emotions such as passion and energy. Green is linked to nature and rebirth, promoting the feeling of renewal and freshness. Yellow is associated with happiness and optimism, while purple can evoke a feeling of mystery and spirituality. Understanding these emotional meanings can help us choose the colors that best suit our emotional needs at any given moment.

The Influence of Colors on Mood: Colorful environments can have a direct impact on our mood and mental health. For example, warm shades like yellow and orange can increase energy and optimism, while cool tones like blue and green can promote calm and reflection. People who suffer from anxiety might benefit from more soothing environments, such as shades of green or blue. Likewise, bright colors can stimulate creativity and enthusiasm.

Color Therapy: Color therapy is a practice that harnesses the power of colors to improve mental well-being. It is based on the theory that exposing a person to specific colors can positively influence their mood and mental health. For example, chromotherapy uses colored lights to treat emotional and physical ailments. The practice of coloring books or drawing with paint can also have calming and therapeutic effects, often used to reduce stress and anxiety.

Incorporating Colors into Everyday Life: There are many ways to harness the benefits of colors in your daily life. We can choose clothes based on our mood or decorate our homes with colors that promote tranquility or productivity. Choosing colorful foods can also impact our mood, as some colors are associated with nutrients beneficial to mental health, such as vitamins and antioxidants.

The connection between colors and mental well-being is a tangible demonstration of how complex and interconnected our inner and outer world is. By consciously harnessing the power of colors, we can modulate our emotions, improve our mood and promote positive mental health. So, the next time we're choosing what to wear, what color to paint a wall, or even what to put on our plate, we might consider how colors affect our mind and spirit.

Chapter 1

Nourishing the Mind and Spirit: The Role of Colors in Foods and Psychological Wellbeing

When it comes to nutrition, we tend to focus primarily on the nutritional values of foods. However, one aspect that is often overlooked is the role that food colors can play in promoting our psychological well-being. The vibrant and varied colors of fruits, vegetables and other foods are not only a feast for the eyes, but can also have beneficial effects on our minds and spirits. In this text, we will explore how food colors affect our psychological well-being and how we can harness this knowledge for better mental health.

The Rainbow on the Plate: Colorful foods provide us with a variety of essential nutrients that contribute to optimal functioning of the body and mind. Each color represents specific groups of beneficial compounds, such as vitamins, minerals, and antioxidants, which not only keep the body healthy but also have a positive impact on the brain. For example, orange foods such as carrots and pumpkins are rich in beta-carotene, which can promote eye health and help improve mood.

Colors and Sensations: Food colors can evoke specific feelings and moods. Red, for example, is often associated with energy and passion. Red fruits such as strawberries and raspberries are rich in antioxidants that can improve blood circulation and boost energy. Green is associated with nature and freshness, and dark green vegetables such as spinach are loaded with folate, which can support mental well-being and reduce the risk of depression.

Foods that Lift Mood: Certain colorful foods can have specific effects on our mood. For example, foods rich in tryptophan, an amino acid precursor of serotonin, the "feel-good neurotransmitter," can promote a positive mood. Bananas, pineapple and avocados, with their warm tones, contain tryptophan and can help improve mood and calmness.

Incorporating Colors into the Diet: A varied diet rich in colors can make a difference to our psychological well-being. Eating a range of colors ensures that we are getting a wide range of beneficial nutrients. For example, a tasty salad with green vegetables, red peppers and orange carrots not only satisfies the palate, but can also nourish our minds with vitamins and antioxidants.

Conclusion: Food colors are not just a visual attraction, but have a tangible impact on our mental health. Each color represents a wealth of nutrients that can support the brain and improve mood. The next time we create a meal, we can consider the power of colors and try to incorporate a variety of hues into our diet. By nourishing our bodies with a range of colors, we can fuel both body and mind for a more balanced and positive life.

And now, with respect to what you have written before, if you can write me another inherent text but more specifically going into the colors of the rainbow

Chapter 2

The Rainbow of Taste and Wellbeing: The Colors of the Rainbow in Food and Mental Health

The rainbow has always been a symbol of beauty and hope. But what might surprise you is that the colors of the rainbow are not only fascinating to the eye, but can also have a profound impact on our mental health. Each color of the rainbow represents a group of unique nutrients and chemicals in foods, which can influence our mood, our vitality and our outlook on life. In this text, we will explore the rainbow colors found in foods and how each can contribute to our psychological well-being.

Red: Passion and Energy Enhancement: The color red evokes feelings of vitality and passion. Foods like strawberries, tomatoes and red peppers are rich in lycopene, a powerful antioxidant that can protect the brain from free radical damage and improve blood circulation. These foods can help increase energy and optimism, contributing to a positive mood.

Orange: Joy and Vitality: The color orange is associated with joy and vitality. Fruits like oranges and peaches are rich in vitamin C, which not only supports the immune system but can also encourage the production of dopamine, the neurotransmitter linked to pleasure and happiness. Eating orange foods can help us feel vibrant and inspired.

Yellow: Optimism and Mental Clarity: Yellow is often linked to optimism and positive energy. Foods like corn and yellow peppers contain carotenoids, which can support eye health and improve memory. Yellow is also associated with mental clarity, helping us to focus and face daily challenges with a positive attitude.

Green: Growth and Renewal: Green is the color of nature and growth. Vegetables like spinach and broccoli are rich in folate and vitamin K, which can support brain health and contribute to cell renewal. Green is also known to promote calm and emotional balance, encouraging reflection and tranquility.

Indigo: Intuition and Balance The color indigo is often associated with intuition and inner balance. Although it is less common in natural foods, some fruits such as blueberries and some varieties of grapes can have indigo hues thanks to the presence of anthocyanins and other beneficial substances. Consuming indigo foods can help you connect with your intuition and promote a sense of mental balance.

Blue: Calm and Serenity: Blue is associated with calm and serenity. Although natural blue foods are rarer, foods like blueberries can provide anthocyanins, which have antioxidant properties and may support brain health. Additionally, exposing your eyes to blue can stimulate the production of melatonin, contributing to better sleep and a rested mind.

Purple: Creativity and Spirituality: Purple is linked to creativity and spirituality. Fruits like grapes and plums are rich in anthocyanins and resveratrol, which can support brain and cardiovascular health. Purple is also associated with internal reflection and the expansion of consciousness, encouraging a deeper perspective on life.

Conclusion: The colors of the rainbow are not only a visual wonder, but are also a guide to a rich and varied diet. Each color represents a unique array of nutrients that can positively influence our mental health. Incorporating a variety of rainbow colors into our diet can help us nourish not only our bodies, but also our minds and spirits. When we eat a rainbow of colors, we can experience an explosion of flavor and an increase in psychological well-being.

Chapter 3

10 recipes with the color Red

1. Red Pepper Risotto:

For how many people: 4

Ingredients:

• 300g of Arborio rice

• 2 red peppers

• 1 onion, finely chopped

• 1 liter of vegetable broth

• 50g of grated parmesan

•	Olive oil

•	Salt and Pepper To Taste.

Method:

1. Grill or roast the red peppers until the skin is black and peels off easily. Peel them, remove the seeds and cut them into strips.

2. In a saucepan, heat some olive oil and fry the onion until translucent.

3. Add the rice and toast it for a couple of minutes.

4. Gradually add the hot vegetable broth, one ladle at a time, stirring continuously until completely cooked (about 18-20 minutes).

5. Add the roasted red peppers and grated parmesan to the risotto. Mix well and serve.

2. Caprese Salad:

For how many people: 2

Ingredients:

• 2 ripe tomatoes

- 200g of buffalo mozzarella

- Fresh basil leaves

- Extra virgin olive oil

- Salt and Pepper To Taste.

Method:

1. Slice the tomatoes and mozzarella and alternate them on a plate.

2. Arrange the basil leaves between the layers of tomato and mozzarella.

3. Season with olive oil, salt and pepper to taste.

3. Arrabbiata Tomato Sauce:

For how many people: 4

Ingredients:

• 400g of peeled tomatoes

• 2 cloves of garlic, finely chopped

• Dried red chili pepper (to taste)

• Olive oil

• Salt and Pepper To Taste.

Method:

1. Heat some olive oil in a pan and add the garlic and dried red chilli.

2. Add the peeled tomatoes and cook over medium-low heat for about 15-20 minutes, mashing the tomatoes with a fork.

3. Season with salt and pepper to taste.

4. Pasta alla Puttanesca:

For how many people: 4

Ingredients:

• 400g of spaghetti

• 400g of peeled tomatoes

• 100g of black olives

• 2 tablespoons of capers

• Red chili pepper (to taste)

• Olive oil

• Salt and Pepper To Taste.

• Fresh parsley (optional)

Method:

1. Cook the spaghetti in plenty of salted water until they are al dente. Drain them and set aside a little cooking water.

2. In a pan, heat some olive oil and add the peeled tomatoes, pitted black olives and capers.

3. Add red chili pepper to taste to give a spicy touch.

4. Cook over medium-low heat for about 10-15 minutes, lightly mashing the tomatoes with a fork.

5. Add the spaghetti to the pan and mix well, adding a little cooking water if necessary.

6. Serve with a drizzle of olive oil and chopped fresh parsley (optional).

5. Gazpacho:

For how many people: 4

Ingredients:

• 6 ripe tomatoes

• 1 red pepper

• 1 cucumber

• 1 clove of garlic

• 1/2 red onion

• 2 tablespoons of red wine vinegar

• 3 tablespoons of olive oil

•   Salt and Pepper To Taste.

Method:

1. Coarsely chop the tomatoes, pepper, cucumber, garlic and onion.

2. Place all ingredients in a high-powered blender and blend until smooth.

3. Add the red wine vinegar, olive oil, salt and pepper. Mix well and leave to cool in the refrigerator for at least an hour before serving.

6. Chicken Cacciatora:

For how many people: 4

Ingredients:

- 4 chicken legs

- 400g of peeled tomatoes

- 1 red pepper

- 1 onion, finely chopped

- 100g of black olives

- 1 glass of red wine

- Olive oil

- Salt and Pepper To Taste.

Method:

1. In a large pot, heat some olive oil and fry the chicken until golden brown on all sides. To put aside.

2. In the same pan, add the onion and the red pepper cut into strips and let them soften.

3. Add the peeled tomatoes and olives. Cook for a few minutes.

4. Add the chicken back to the pot and pour in the red wine. Allow the alcohol to evaporate.

5. Cover and cook on low heat for about 30-40 minutes, or until the chicken is cooked through.

7. Red Pepper Cream:

For how many people: 4

Ingredients:

- 4 red peppers

- 2 medium potatoes

- 1 liter of vegetable broth

- 100ml of cream

- Olive oil

- Salt and Pepper To Taste.

Method:

1. Grill or roast the red peppers until the skin is black and peels off easily. Peel them, remove the seeds and cut them into pieces.

2. Peel and cut the potatoes into cubes.

3. In a saucepan, heat some olive oil and add the peppers and potatoes. Cook for a few minutes.

4. Add the vegetable broth and cook until the potatoes are soft.

5. Blend everything until you obtain a smooth cream, adding the cream. Season with salt and pepper.

8. Spaghetti all'Amatriciana:

For how many people: 4

Ingredients:

- 400g of spaghetti

- 150g of bacon or bacon, diced

- 400g of peeled tomatoes

- Dried red chili pepper (to taste)

- 50g of grated pecorino romano

- Olive oil

- Salt and Pepper To Taste.

Method:

1. Cook the spaghetti in plenty of salted water until cooked tooth. Drain them and set aside a little cooking water.

2. In a pan, heat some olive oil and add the bacon or bacon. Brown them well.

3. Add the peeled tomatoes and dried red chili pepper to taste. Cook over medium-low heat for about 10-15 minutes.

4. Add the spaghetti to the pan and mix well, adding a little cooking water if necessary.

5. Serve with plenty of grated pecorino romano.

9. Roasted Red Pepper Sauce:

For how many people: 4

Ingredients:

- 2 red peppers

- 2 cloves of garlic

- 3 tablespoons of olive oil

- 1 tablespoon red wine vinegar

- Salt and Pepper To Taste.

Method:

1. Grill or roast the red peppers until the skin is black and peels off easily. Peel them, remove the seeds and cut them into strips.

2. Place the roasted peppers in a blender with the garlic, olive oil, and red wine vinegar.

3. Blend until smooth. Season with salt and pepper.

10. Chocolate and Raspberry Cake:

For how many people: 8

Ingredients:

- 200g of dark chocolate

- 150g of fresh raspberries

- 4 eggs

- 150g of butter

- 150g of sugar

- 100g of flour

- 1 sachet of baking powder

Method:

1. Melt the dark chocolate in a bain-marie or in the microwave and let it cool slightly.

2. In the meantime, beat the eggs with the sugar until the mixture becomes frothy. Add the melted chocolate and mix well.

3. Add the sifted flour with the yeast and mix until a homogeneous mixture is obtained.

4. Gently fold in the raspberries.

5. Pour the mixture into a buttered and floured pan and bake in a pre-heated oven at 180°C for approximately 30-35 minutes, or until the cake is well cooked.

Chapter 4

10 recipes with the color Orange

1. Curry Pumpkin Soup:

• Servings: 4

•   Ingredients:

• 500g of pumpkin, cut into cubes

• 400ml of coconut milk

• 1 onion, chopped

• 2 teaspoons curry powder

• 2 cloves of garlic, minced

• 2 tablespoons of olive oil

• Salt and pepper to taste

- Method:

1. In a saucepan, heat the olive oil and cook the onion and garlic until golden.

2. Add pumpkin and curry powder, mix well.

3. Add the coconut milk and cook over medium-low heat until the squash is soft.

4. Blend the soup until smooth. Season with salt and pepper.

2. Pumpkin and Gorgonzola Risotto:

- Servings: 4

- Ingredients:

- 300g of Arborio rice

- 300g of pumpkin, cut into cubes

- 100g of gorgonzola

- 1 onion, chopped

- 1 liter of vegetable broth

- 2 tablespoons butter

- 2 tablespoons of olive oil

- Salt and pepper to taste

- Method:

1. In a saucepan, heat the olive oil and cook the onion until transparent.

2. Add the pumpkin and rice and toast them for a couple of minutes.

3. Gradually add the vegetable broth, stirring occasionally, until the rice is cooked.

4. Turn off the heat, add the gorgonzola and butter. Mix well and serve.

3. Roasted Chicken with Sweet Potatoes:

• Servings: 4

•   Ingredients:

• 4 chicken breasts

• 4 sweet potatoes, cut into cubes

• 4 cloves of garlic, minced

• Fresh rosemary sprigs

•   Olive oil

• Salt and pepper to taste

•   Method:

1. Preheat the oven to 200°C.

2. Place the chicken and potatoes on a baking tray. Season with olive oil, garlic, rosemary, salt and pepper.

3. Bake in the oven for about 40-45 minutes or until the chicken is golden brown and the potatoes are soft.

4. Carrot and Ginger Sauce:

• Servings: 4

•	Ingredients:

• 300g of carrots, cut into rounds

• 2 tablespoons fresh ginger, grated

• 2 cloves of garlic, minced

- 2 tablespoons of olive oil

- Salt and pepper to taste

-     Method:

1. Cook carrots in boiling water until tender.

2. Drain the carrots and place them in a blender with the garlic, ginger, olive oil, salt and pepper.

3. Blend until you obtain a smooth sauce.

5. Carrot and Orange Salad:

- Servings: 4

-     Ingredients:

- 300g carrots, grated

- 2 oranges, peeled and cut into wedges

- 50g of almonds, toasted and chopped

- Fresh parsley, chopped

- Lemon juice

- Olive oil

- Salt and pepper to taste

- Method:

1. In a bowl, mix the grated carrots, orange segments, almonds and parsley.

2. Season with lemon juice, olive oil, salt and pepper.

6. Pasta with Pumpkin and Sage:

- Servings: 4

- Ingredients:

- 300g of pasta (preferably gnocchi or tagliatelle)

- 300g of pumpkin, cut into cubes

- 50g of butter

- Fresh sage leaves

- Grated Parmesan cheese

- Salt and pepper to taste

- Method:

1. Steam the pumpkin until soft. Mash it with a fork to obtain a puree.

2. In a pan, melt the butter and add the sage leaves. Let them brown.

3. Cook the pasta al dente. Drain it and add it to the pan with the butter and sage.

4. Add the pumpkin puree and mix well. Season with parmesan, salt and pepper.

7. Salmon and Saffron Risotto:

- Servings: 4

- Ingredients:

- 300g of Arborio rice

- 200g of salmon, cut into cubes

- Saffron in pistils or powder

- 1 onion, chopped

- 1 liter of fish broth

- 2 tablespoons butter

- 2 tablespoons of olive oil

- Salt and pepper to taste

- Method:

1. In a saucepan, heat the olive oil and cook the onion until transparent.

2. Add the rice and toast it for a couple of minutes.

3. Gradually add the fish broth, stirring occasionally, until the rice is cooked.

4. Add the salmon and saffron, mix well. Season with salt and pepper.

8. Watermelon and Carrot Smoothie:

- Servings: 2

- Ingredients:

• 2 cups watermelon, cut into cubes

• 1 cup carrots, cut into rounds

• 1 tablespoon fresh ginger, grated

• Juice of half a lemon

• Honey to taste

- Method:

1. Place the watermelon, carrots and ginger into the blender.

2. Add the lemon juice and blend until smooth.

3. Add honey if desired and mix well.

9. Carrot and Almond Cake:

- Servings: 6

- Ingredients:

- 300g carrots, grated

- 150g of chopped almonds

- 4 eggs

- 100g of sugar

- 100g of flour

- 1 sachet of yeast

- 1 teaspoon of ground cinnamon

- A pinch of salt

- Method:

1. In a bowl, mix the grated carrots and chopped almonds.

2. In another bowl, beat the eggs with the sugar until the mixture becomes frothy.

3. Add the flour, baking powder, cinnamon and salt to the egg mixture and mix well.

4. Add the carrot and almond mixture to the dough and mix gently.

5. Pour the dough i n a cake tin and bake in a preheated oven at 180°C for around 35-40 minutes.

10. Peach and Mango Ice Cream:

Servings: 4

Ingredients: - 2 ripe peaches - 1 ripe mango - 100g of sugar - 200ml of fresh cream - 100ml of milk - Juice of half a lemon

- Method:

- 1. Peel and cut the peaches and mango into pieces.

  2. Place the fruit in the blender with the sugar and lemon juice. Blend until you obtain a smooth puree.

  3. In another bowl, whip fresh cream until soft peaks form.

  4. Gently mix the fruit puree with the whipped cream and milk.

  5. Pour the mixture into a sorbet maker and follow the manufacturer's instructions to prepare the ice cream.place into a sorbet

maker and follow the manufacturer's instructions to prepare the ice cream.

Chapter 5

10 recipes with the color Yellow

1. Saffron risotto

For: 4 people

Ingredients:

- 320g of rice

- 1 sachet of saffron

- 1 onion

- 1 liter of vegetable broth

- 50g of butter

- 60g of grated Parmesan

- Salt and Pepper To Taste.

Method:

1. Prepare the vegetable broth and dissolve the saffron sachet in a little hot broth.

2. In a pan, fry the chopped onion in the butter until it becomes transparent.

3. Add the rice and toast it for a couple of minutes, mixing well.

4. Pour a ladle of hot broth into the pan and stir until the liquid is absorbed.

5. Continue adding the broth by the ladleful, stirring occasionally, until the rice is cooked al dente.

6. Add the dissolved saffron and grated Parmesan, mix well.

7. Let it rest for a minute and then serve.

2. Chicken Curry

For: 4 people

Ingredients:

- 500g of chicken breast

- 2 tablespoons curry powder

- 1 onion

- 2 cloves of garlic

- 1 yellow pepper

- 400ml of coconut milk

- Olive oil

- Salt and Pepper To Taste.

Method:

1. Dice the chicken breast and sprinkle with curry powder.

2. In a pan, heat the olive oil and cook the chicken until golden. Set it aside.

3. In the same pan, add a little oil if necessary and fry the chopped onion and garlic until translucent.

4. Add the yellow pepper in thin strips and cook for a few minutes.

5. Add the chicken to the pan and pour in the coconut milk. Cook for about 10-15 minutes over medium-low heat.

6. Serve with white or basmati rice.

3. Yellow Pepper Omelette

For 2 people

Ingredients:

- 4 eggs

- 1 yellow pepper

- 1 onion

- Salt and Pepper To Taste.

- Olive oil

Method:

1. Cut the pepper into cubes and the onion into thin slices.

2. In a pan, heat some olive oil and fry the pepper and onion until soft.

3. In a bowl, beat the eggs with salt and pepper.

4. Pour the beaten eggs into the pan with the vegetables and cook over medium-high heat until the omelette is well set.

5. Serve hot or at room temperature.

4. Creamed Corn

For: 4 people

Ingredients:

- 4 ears of corn

- 1 potato

- 1 onion

- 1 liter of vegetable broth

- 50g of butter

- Salt and Pepper To Taste.

- Chopped parsley for garnish

Method:

1. Remove the corn kernels from the ears.

2. In a saucepan, melt the butter and fry the chopped onion until transparent.

3. Add the diced potato and corn kernels. Fry for a few minutes.

4. Add the vegetable broth and cook until the vegetables are tender.

5. Blend everything until you obtain a smooth cream.

6. Season with salt and pepper and garnish with chopped parsley.

5. Pumpkin puree

For: 4 people

Ingredients:

• 800g of pumpkin

• 2 potatoes

• 1 onion

• 1 liter of vegetable broth

- 50g of butter

- Nutmeg

- Salt and Pepper To Taste.

Method:

1. Cut the pumpkin and potatoes into large pieces.

2. In a saucepan, melt the butter and fry the chopped onion until transparent.

3. Add the pumpkin and potatoes and cook for a few minutes.

4. Pour in the vegetable broth and cook until the vegetables are soft.

5. Blend everything until you get a smooth puree.

6. Season with salt, pepper and nutmeg.

6. Curry Sauce for Pasta

For: 4 people

Ingredients:

- 1 yellow pepper

- 1 onion

- 2 cloves of garlic

- 200ml of cream

- 2 tablespoons curry powder

- Olive oil

- Salt and Pepper To Taste.

Method:

1. Dice the pepper, chop the onion and garlic finely.

2. In a pan, heat some olive oil and fry the onion and garlic until golden.

3. Add the pepper and cook until soft.

4. Add curry powder and mix well.

5. Pour in the cream and cook for a few minutes until the sauce is well blended.

6. Season with salt and pepper and serve with the pasta cooked al dente.

7. Peppers Stuffed with Rice

For: 4 people

Ingredients:

- 4 yellow peppers

- 200g of rice

- 1 onion

- 2 cloves of garlic

- 200g of peeled tomatoes

- 100g of grated cheese

- Olive oil

- Salt and Pepper To Taste.

Method:

1. Cook the rice according to the package instructions.

2. Cut the tops of the peppers, remove the seeds and internal membranes.

3. In a pan, heat some olive oil and fry the chopped onion and garlic until golden.

4. Add the peeled tomatoes and cook for a few minutes.

5. Add the cooked rice and mix well.

6. Fill the peppers with the rice mixture and place them on a baking tray.

7. Sprinkle with grated cheese and cook in the oven at 180°C for about 20-25 minutes.

8. Corn and Bean Salad

For: 4 people

Ingredients:

• 200g of canned corn

- 200g of canned cannellini beans

- 1 yellow pepper

- 1 red onion

- 1 lemon (juice)

- 2 tablespoons of olive oil

- Chopped fresh parsley

- Salt and Pepper To Taste.

Method:

1. Drain and rinse the corn and beans well.

2. Cut the pepper diced and the onion thinly sliced.

3. In a large bowl, combine corn, beans, bell pepper, and onion.

4. Squeeze the lemon juice and add the olive oil, salt and pepper. Mix well.

5. Sprinkle with chopped fresh parsley before serving.

9. Apricot tart

For: 8 people

Ingredients:

- 250g of flour

- 125g of butter

- 1 egg

- 100g of sugar

- 500g of apricots

- Powdered sugar

Method:

1. Prepare the shortcrust pastry by mixing the flour, butter, egg and sugar. Form a ball and let it rest in the refrigerator for at least 30 minutes.

2. Roll out the shortcrust pastry and line a tart pan with it.

3. Arrange the halved apricots on the pasta.

4. Dust with icing sugar and bake in the oven at 180°C for about 30-40 minutes.

10. Banana Ice Cream

For: 4 people

Ingredients:

- 4 ripe bananas

- 200ml of Greek yogurt

- 50g of sugar

- Lemon juice

Method:

1. Cut the bananas into slices and place them in the freezer for at least 2 hours.

2. Blend the bananas with the Greek yogurt, sugar and lemon juice until you obtain a creamy consistency.

3. Transfer the mixture into a container and place it back in the freezer for at least 2 hours, stirring every half hour

Chapter 6

10 recipes with the color Green

1. Spinach and Strawberry Salad

For 4 people:

Ingredients:

- 200g of fresh spinach

- 200g of strawberries

- 50g of walnuts

- 50g of goat's cheese

- Olive oil

- Balsamic vinegar

- Salt and pepper

Method:

1. Wash and dry the spinach and strawberries.

2. Cut the strawberries into thin slices and chop the walnuts.

3. In a large bowl, mix the spinach, strawberries and walnuts.

4. Crumble the goat cheese over the salad.

5. Season with olive oil, balsamic vinegar, salt and pepper to taste.

2. Pasta with Basil Pesto

For 4 people:

Ingredients:

• 400g of pasta (preferably trofie or linguine)

- 2 bunches of fresh basil

- 50g of pine nuts

- 2 cloves of garlic

- 100g of grated Parmigiano Reggiano

- 100ml of extra virgin olive oil

- Salt and pepper

Method:

1. Cook the pasta in plenty of salted water following the instructions on the package.

2. In the meantime, prepare the pesto. In a blender, combine basil, pine nuts, garlic, Parmigiano Reggiano and olive oil. Blend until you obtain a smooth consistency.

3. Drain the pasta al dente and season it with the pesto.

4. Mix well and serve hot.

3. Pea Soup

For 4 people:

Ingredients:

• 400g of fresh or frozen peas

• 1 onion

• 1 potato

• 1 carrot

• 1 liter of vegetable broth

- Olive oil

- Salt and pepper

• Fresh parsley (for garnish)

Method:

1. Finely chop the onion and cut the potato and carrot into cubes.

2. In a saucepan, fry the onion in a little olive oil until translucent.

3. Add the peas, potato and carrot. Mix for a couple of minutes.

4. Pour in the vegetable broth and bring to the boil.

5. Reduce the heat and cook over medium-low heat for about 20-25 minutes or until the vegetables are tender.

6. Blend the soup until you obtain a velvety consistency.

7. Season with salt and pepper. Serve garnished with fresh parsley.

4. Asparagus risotto

For 4 people:

Ingredients:

• 300g of Arborio rice

• 300g of green asparagus

• 1 onion

- 1 liter of vegetable broth

- 60g of butter

- 60g of grated Parmigiano Reggiano

- Salt and pepper

Method:

1. Clean the asparagus and cut them into small pieces. Steam them until tender but still crunchy.

2. In a saucepan, fry the chopped onion in half the butter until translucent.

3. Add the rice and toast it for a couple of minutes.

4. Gradually add the vegetable broth, one ladle at a time, stirring continuously and

waiting for it to be absorbed before adding more.

5. When the rice is almost cooked, add the asparagus and continue cooking until the risotto reaches the desired consistency.

6. Turn off the heat, add the rest of the butter and the Parmigiano Reggiano. Mix well and serve.

5. Courgette and Pea Omelette

For 4 people:

Ingredients:

- 6 eggs

- 2 medium courgettes

- 100g of fresh or frozen peas

- 50g of grated cheese (of your choice)

- Olive oil

- Salt and pepper

Method:

1. Chop the courgettes and cook them in a pan with a little olive oil until soft.

2. Add the peas and cook for another 2-3 minutes.

3. In a bowl, beat the eggs and add the grated cheese, salt and pepper to taste.

4. Pour the eggs into the pan with the courgettes and peas.

5. Cook over medium-low heat until the omelette sets around the edges.

6. Place the pan in a pre-heated oven at 180°C for about 5 minutes or until the omelette is completely cooked.

7. Serve hot or at room temperature.

6. Quinoa, Avocado and Chickpea Salad

For 4 people:

Ingredients:

• 1 cup quinoa

• 2 cups of water

- 1 ripe avocado

- 1 can chickpeas, rinsed and drained

- 1 cucumber

- 1 lemon (juice)

- 2 tablespoons of olive oil

- 50g of feta (optional)

- Salt and pepper

- Fresh mint leaves (optional)

Method:

1. Rinse the quinoa well under running water.

2. In a saucepan, bring 2 cups of water to a boil, add the quinoa and cook over low heat

for 15 to 20 minutes or until the water is absorbed and the quinoa is cooked. Let cool.

3. Cut the avocado into cubes, the cucumber into thin slices and place them in a large bowl. Add the chickpeas.

4. Add the lemon juice, olive oil, salt and pepper, and mix well.

5. Add the cooled quinoa and mix again.

6. If desired, add crumbled feta and fresh mint leaves to taste.

7. Let it rest in the refrigerator for at least 30 minutes before serving.

7. Spinach Pesto Risotto

For 4 people:

Ingredients:

- 300g of Arborio rice

- 200g of fresh spinach

- 50g of pine nuts

- 2 cloves of garlic

- 60g of grated Parmigiano Reggiano

- 60ml of olive oil

- Salt and pepper

Method:

1. Prepare the spinach pesto: in a blender, combine the spinach, pine nuts, garlic, l

Parmigiano Reggiano and olive oil. Blend until you obtain a smooth consistency.

2. In a pan, toast the rice for a couple of minutes.

3. Gradually add the vegetable broth, one ladle at a time, stirring continuously and waiting for it to be absorbed before adding more.

4. When the rice is almost cooked, add the spinach pesto and mix well.

5. Continue cooking until the risotto reaches the desired consistency. Season with salt and pepper.

8. Broccoli and Potato Soup

For 4 people:

Ingredients:

- 500g of broccoli

- 2 medium potatoes

- 1 onion

- 1 liter of vegetable broth

- Olive oil

- Salt and pepper

Method:

1. Cut the broccoli into florets and the potatoes into cubes.

2. In a pan, fry the chopped onion in a little olive oil until translucent.

3. Add the broccoli and potatoes and mix for a couple of minutes.

4. Pour in the vegetable broth and bring to the boil.

5. Reduce the heat and cook over medium-low heat for about 20-25 minutes or until the vegetables are tender.

6. Blend the soup until you obtain a velvety consistency. Season with salt and pepper.

9. Avocado and Black Bean Salad

For 4 people:

Ingredients:

- 2 avocados

- 400g canned black beans, rinsed and drained

- 1 tomato

- 1 red onion

- Juice of 2 lemons

- 2 tablespoons of olive oil

- Fresh coriander (optional)

- Salt and pepper

Method:

1. Cut the avocados into cubes and place them in a large bowl.

2. Add the black beans, diced tomato and thinly sliced red onion.

3. In a small bowl, mix the lemon juice, olive oil, salt and pepper. Pour over salad and mix well.

4. If you prefer, garnish with fresh coriander.

10. Pasta with Salmon and Peas

For 4 people:

Ingredients:

• 400g of pasta (preferably penne or farfalle)

• 200g of smoked salmon

• 200g of fresh or frozen peas

• 200ml of cooking cream

• 2 tablespoons butter

- Salt and pepper

Method:

1. Cook the pasta in plenty of salted water following the instructions on the package.

2. In the meantime, cut the salmon into strips and cook the peas in boiling water for a few minutes.

3. In a pan, melt the butter and add the salmon. Cook for 2-3 minutes.

4. Add the peas and cream. Cook over medium heat until the cream is slightly reduced.

5. Drain the pasta and add it to the pan with the salmon and peas. Mix well and serve.

Chapter 7

10 recipes with the color Purple

1. Risotto with aubergines and radicchio (4 people)

Ingredients:

- 320g of arborio rice

- 2 medium aubergines

- 1 head of red radicchio

- 1 onion

- 1 clove of garlic

- Vegetable broth to taste

- Olive oil

- Salt and Pepper To Taste.

- Grated parmesan cheese (optional)

Method:

1. Cut the aubergines into cubes and cook them in a pan with olive oil until they become soft and golden.

2. In a saucepan, fry the chopped onion and garlic in olive oil. Add the rice and toast it for a few minutes.

3. Add the radicchio cut into thin strips and continue to cook, stirring, until it softens.

4. Gradually pour in the hot broth and continue cooking, stirring occasionally.

5. When the rice is almost ready, add the eggplant and stir in cheese (if desired). Season with salt and pepper.

2. Purple potato cream (4 people)

Ingredients:

• 500g of purple potatoes

• 1 onion

• 2 cloves of garlic

• 1 liter of vegetable broth

• 100ml of fresh cream

•   Salt and Pepper To Taste.

• Chopped parsley (for garnish)

Method:

1. Peel and cut the potatoes into cubes.

2. In a saucepan, fry the chopped onion and garlic in olive oil. Add the potatoes and vegetable broth.

3. Cook until potatoes are tender.

4. Blend with an immersion blender until you obtain a creamy consistency.

5. Add the fresh cream, season with salt and pepper, and mix well.

6. Serve with chopped parsley as a garnish.

3. Red Cabbage and Raisin Salad (4 servings)

Ingredients:

• 1 small red cabbage

• 50g of raisins

• 50g of walnuts

• Olive oil

• Lemon juice

• Salt and Pepper To Taste.

Method:

1. Finely slice the red cabbage and place it in a large bowl.

2. Soak the raisins in hot water for about 10 minutes, then drain them and add them to the cabbage.

3. Coarsely chop the walnuts and add them to the salad.

4. Season with olive oil, lemon juice, salt and pepper to taste. Mix well.

4. Spaghetti with beetroot pesto (4 people)

Ingredients:

- 400g of spaghetti

- 2 medium beets

- 50g of walnuts

- 50g of grated parmesan cheese

- 2 cloves of garlic

- Olive oil

- Salt and Pepper To Taste.

Method:

1. Boil the beets, peel them and cut them into pieces.

2. Blend the beets with the walnuts, cheese, garlic and a drizzle of olive oil until smooth.

3. Cook the spaghetti in salted water, drain them and mix them with the beetroot pesto.

4. Add salt and pepper to taste.

5. Purple potato flan (6 people)

Ingredients:

- 800g of purple potatoes

- 100ml of milk

- 50g of butter

- 2 eggs

- 100g of grated cheese

- Salt and Pepper To Taste.

- Nutmeg (optional)

Method:

1. Peel, cut and cook the potatoes in salted water until tender. Drain them and pass them through a potato masher.

2. Heat the milk with the butter until the butter melts completely.

3. Add the milk and grated cheese to the mashed potatoes and mix well. Season with salt, pepper and nutmeg (if desired).

4. Add the beaten eggs and mix again.

5. Pour the mixture into a buttered pan and bake it at 180°C for about 30-40 minutes, until it is golden brown.

6. Purple Cauliflower Soup (4 servings)

Ingredients:

- 1 medium purple cauliflower

- 1 onion

- 2 medium potatoes

- 1 liter of vegetable broth

- 100ml of fresh cream

- Olive oil

- Salt and Pepper To Taste.

- Fresh thyme (for garnish)

Method:

1. Peel and chop the onion. Cut the potatoes and cauliflower into pieces.

2. In a saucepan, sauté the onion in olive oil until translucent.

3. Add the potatoes and cauliflower and cook for a few minutes, stirring.

4. Pour in the vegetable broth and cook until the vegetables are tender.

5. Blend the soup with an immersion blender until smooth.

6. Add the fresh cream, season with salt and pepper, and mix well.

7. Serve with fresh thyme leaves as garnish.

7. Lavender panna cotta (4 people)

Ingredients:

• 500ml of fresh cream

• 100g of sugar

* 2 tablespoons dried lavender flowers

* 4 gelatin sheets

* 100ml of milk

Method:

1. Place the lavender flowers in a bowl with the cream and leave them to infuse at room temperature for at least 2 hours.

2. Heat the milk and dissolve the gelatin in it.

3. Heat the cream with the lavender flowers over low heat, without letting it boil. Strain the cream to remove the flowers.

4. Mix the cream, milk with gelatin and sugar.

5. Pour the mixture into molds and place in the refrigerator for at least 4 hours, or until it solidifies completely.

8. Raisin and currant muffins (12 muffins)

Ingredients:

• 200g of flour

• 100g of sugar

• 1 sachet of baking powder

•   2 eggs

• 100ml of milk

• 100g of melted butter

• 100g of raisins

• 100g of currants

Method:

1. In a bowl, mix the flour, sugar and baking powder.

2. In another bowl, beat the eggs, add add milk and melted butter.

3. Pour the liquid mixture into the bowl with the dry ingredients and mix briefly.

4. Add the raisins and currants and mix gently.

5. Distribute the mixture into the muffin cups and bake in a preheated oven at 180°C for approximately 20-25 minutes, or until the muffins are golden.

9. Aubergine and currant ice cream (4 people)

Ingredients:

- 2 medium aubergines

- 100g of currants

- 100g of sugar

- 250ml of fresh cream

- 100ml of milk

Method:

1. Bake the aubergines in the oven until soft. Peel them and blend the pulp.

2. In a saucepan, dissolve the sugar in a little water until you get a syrup.

3. Mix the aubergine pulp, syrup, milk and fresh cream.

4. Add the currants and pour the mixture into the ice cream maker.

5. Process the ice cream according to your ice cream maker's instructions, then transfer it to an airtight container and place it in the freezer for at least 4 hours.

10. Blackberry and lavender cake (8 people)

Ingredients:

• 200g of blackberries

- 2 tablespoons dried lavender flowers

- 200g of flour

- 150g of sugar

- 150g of butter

- 3 eggs

- 1 sachet of baking powder

Method:

1. In a bowl, mix the flour and baking powder.

2. In another bowl, beat the butter with the sugar until you get a frothy mixture. Add the eggs, one at a time.

3. Gradually fold the dry ingredients into the butter and egg mixture.

4. Add the lavender flowers and blackberries (reserve some for decoration) and mix gently.

5. Pour the mixture into a buttered cake tin and bake in a preheated oven at 180°C for about 40-45 minutes, or until the cake is golden.

6. Decorate it with the remaining blackberries and lavender flowers.

Chapter 8

10 recipes with the color Blue and Indigo

1. Spirulina Algae Pancakes

For 2 people:

Ingredients:

• 1 cup flour

• 1 cup of milk

• 1 egg

• 2 tablespoons of sugar

• 1 tablespoon of oil

• 1 teaspoon of spirulina algae powder

Method:

1. In a bowl, mix the flour, milk, egg, sugar and oil until smooth.

2. Add the spirulina algae and mix well until the color is uniform.

3. Heat a non-stick pan and cook the pancakes on both sides until golden.

2. Purple Potato Salad

For 4 people:

Ingredients:

- 4 purple potatoes

- 1/2 cup mayonnaise

- 2 tablespoons Dijon mustard

- 1/4 cup chopped red onion

- 2 tablespoons chopped fresh parsley

- Salt and Pepper To Taste.

Method:

1. Cook the potatoes in salted water until tender. Drain them and let them cool.

2. Cut the potatoes into cubes and place them in a large bowl.

3. In another bowl, mix the mayonnaise, mustard, red onion, parsley, salt and pepper.

4. Pour the mixture over the potatoes and toss gently until well seasoned.

3. Blue Sushi with Black Rice and Spirulina

For 2 people:

Ingredients:

- 1 cup black rice

- 2 sheets of nori seaweed

- 1 teaspoon of spirulina algae powder

• Fish of your choice (salmon, tuna, avocado, etc.)

• Rice vinegar, soy sauce and pickled ginger to accompany

Method:

1. Cook the black rice according to the package instructions and let it cool.

2. Mix the spirulina algae with the cooked rice until it turns a uniform blue color.

3. Spread the rice on the nori sheet, leaving free space around the edges.

4. Add the fish or avocado to the center of the rice.

5. Roll the nori seaweed with the filling and cut the roll into pieces.

4. Blue Pizza with Purple Potatoes and Goat Cheese

For 2 people:

Ingredients:

- 1 pizza base

- 2 purple potatoes, thinly sliced

- 100g of goat's cheese

- Black olives (optional)

- Fresh rosemary

- Olive oil

Method:

1. Spread the pizza dough on a baking tray.

2. Brush with olive oil and bake in a pre-heated oven following package instructions.

3. Meanwhile, cook the potatoes in salted water until tender, then drain.

4. Spread the potatoes over the cooked pizza, add the goat cheese and olives.

5. Return to the oven until the cheese begins to melt.

6. Sprinkle with fresh rosemary before serving.

5. Orange and Spirulina Smoothie

For 2 people:

Ingredients:

• 2 oranges

• 1 teaspoon of spirulina algae powder

• 1 banana

• 1/2 cup Greek yogurt

• Honey to taste

Method:

1. Squeeze the juice from the oranges and pour it into the blender.

2. Add the banana, Greek yogurt, spirulina and honey.

3. Blend until smooth.

6. Blueberry Ice Cream

For 4 people:

Ingredients:

• 2 cups fresh or frozen blueberries

• 1/2 cup milk

• 1/4 cup sugar

• 1 teaspoon vanilla extract

Method:

1. Place blueberries, milk, sugar and vanilla extract in a high-powered blender.

2. Blend until smooth.

3. Transfer the mixture to a sorbet maker and follow the manufacturer's instructions.

4. Freeze the ice cream for about an hour before serving.

7. Buckwheat Spaghetti with Spirulina Pesto

For 2 people:

Ingredients:

- 200g of buckwheat spaghetti

- 1 teaspoon of spirulina algae powder

- 1 cup fresh basil leaves

- 1/4 cup pine nuts

- 1/4 cup grated Parmesan cheese

- 1 clove of garlic

- Extra virgin olive oil

Method:

1. Cook the spaghetti in salted water until al dente, then drain.

2. Meanwhile, blend the basil, pine nuts, parmesan cheese, garlic and olive oil until you have a pesto.

3. Add the spirulina to the pesto and mix well.

4. Season the spaghetti with pesto and mix gently.

8. Chia Pudding with Blueberries

For 2 people:

Ingredients:

- 1/4 cup chia seeds

- 1 cup coconut milk

- 1 tablespoon honey

- 1/4 cup fresh blueberries

Method:

1. Mix chia seeds, coconut milk and honey in a bowl.

2. Cover and refrigerate for at least 2 hours or overnight.

3. Stir again before serving and garnish with fresh blueberries.

9. Indigo risotto with prawns and saffron

For 4 people:

Ingredients:

• 300g of Arborio rice

• 400g of peeled prawns

• 1 onion finely chopped

• 2 cloves of garlic, chopped

• 1 cup of white wine

• 1 liter of vegetable broth

• 1 sachet of saffron powder

• 2 tablespoons butter

• Extra virgin olive oil

- Salt and Pepper To Taste.

• Grated parmesan cheese (optional)

Method:

1. Bring the vegetable broth to the boil in a saucepan and keep it warm over low heat.

2. In a large pan , heat some olive oil and add the onion and garlic. Fry until they become translucent.

3. Add the rice and toast it for a couple of minutes, stirring constantly.

4. Pour in the white wine and let it evaporate completely.

5. Add the saffron and a ladle of hot broth to the rice. Continue to cook over medium-low

heat, stirring regularly and adding stock as it is absorbed.

6. Meanwhile, in another pan, heat some olive oil and cook the prawns until pink and fully cooked.

7. Add the prawns to the risotto about halfway through cooking.

8. Continue adding stock and stirring until risotto reaches desired consistency (about 18-20 minutes total).

9. Mix the risotto with the butter and, if desired, add the grated Parmesan cheese.

10. Serve the risotto hot, garnished with a few extra prawns and a sprinkling of saffron for a stunning presentation.

10. Orange and Blueberry Muffins

For 6 muffins:

Ingredients:

- 1 1/2 cups flour

- 1/2 cup sugar

- 2 teaspoons of baking powder

- 1/2 teaspoon salt

- 1/2 cup milk

- 1/4 cup vegetable oil

- 1 egg

- Grated orange zest

- 1/2 cup blueberries

Method:

1. Preheat the oven to 180°C and prepare a muffin tray with paper liners.

2. In a bowl, mix the flour, sugar, baking powder and salt.

3. In another bowl, mix the milk, oil, egg and orange zest.

4. Combine the wet ingredients with the dry ones and mix slightly.

5. Add the blueberries and mix gently.

6. Fill the cups 2/3 full and bake in the oven for about 20-25 minutes or until golden.

Index

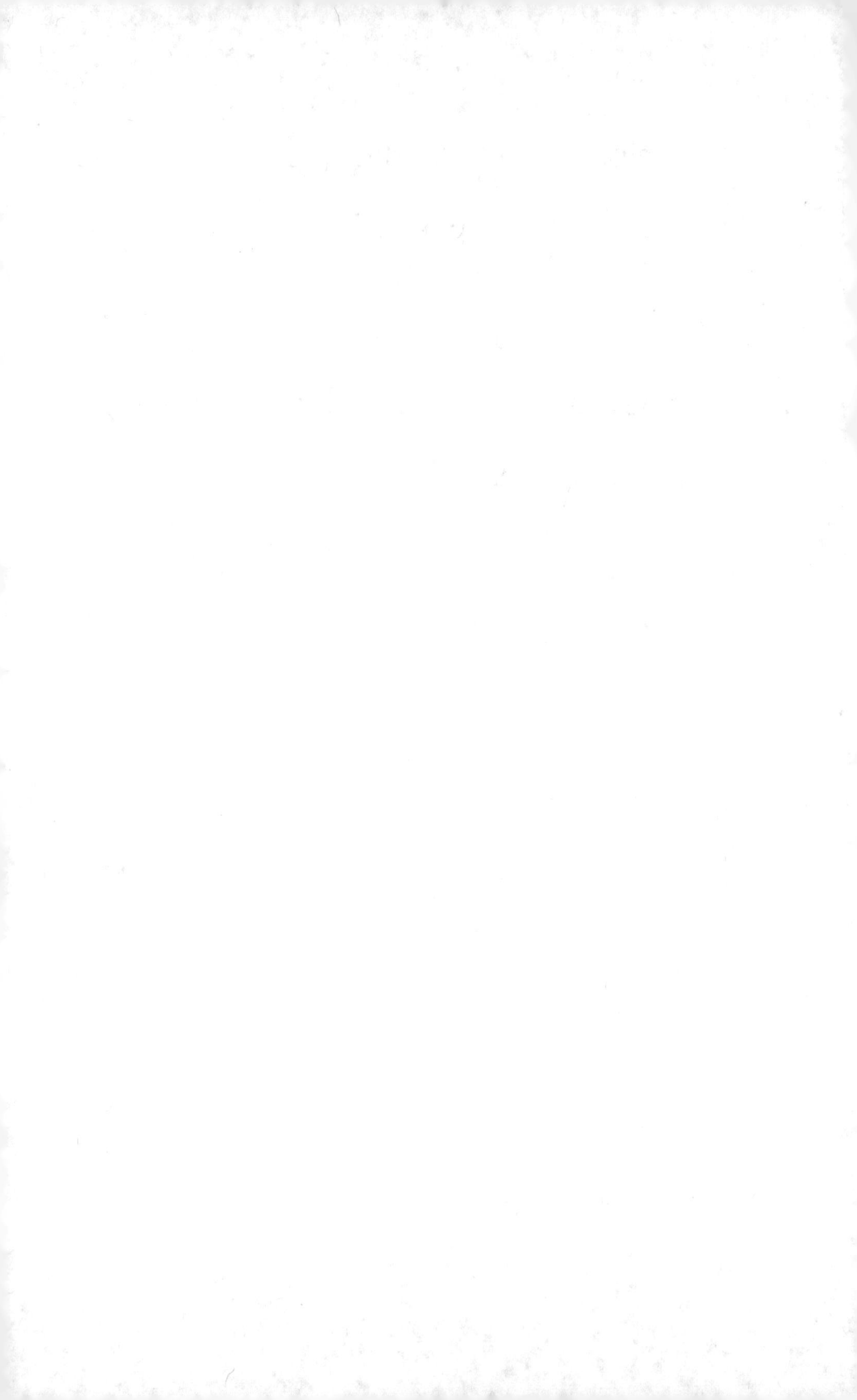

www.ingramcontent.com/pod-product-compliance
Lightning Source LLC
Chambersburg PA
CBHW070808260726
48660CB00005B/1761